Ollyaga
You are Special!

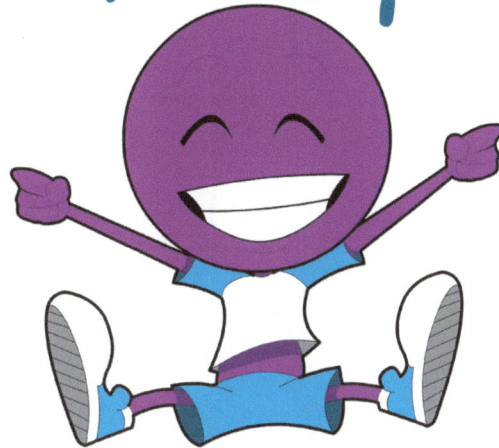

HOLYCOW
BOOK PUBLISHERS

One day
I asked some of my friends,
"What makes you
Special?"

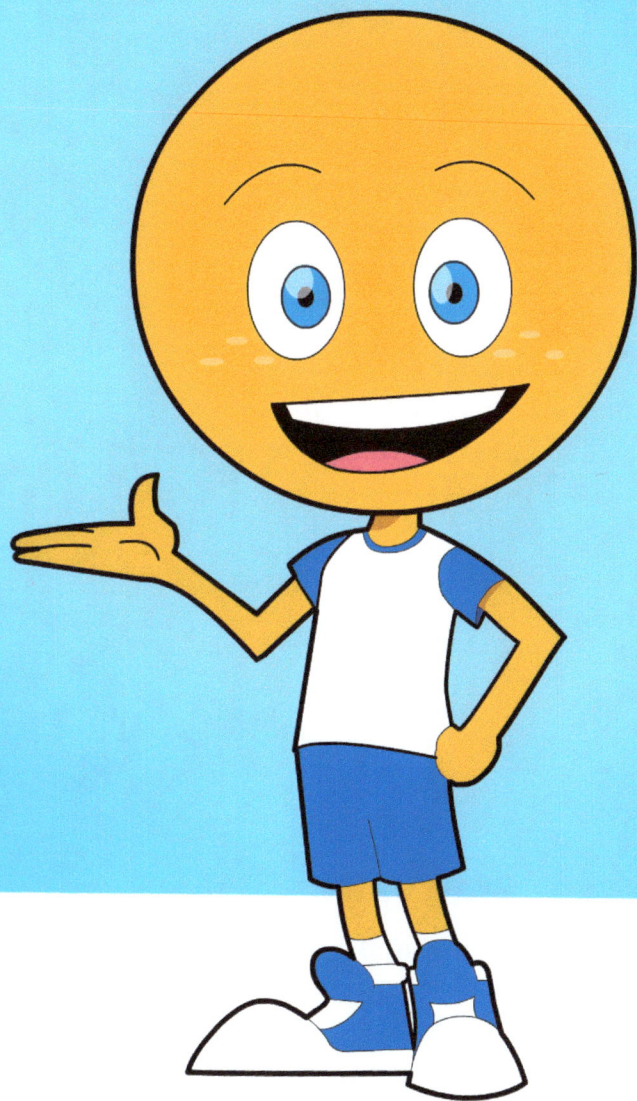

Adam said, "I am special because I can draw!"

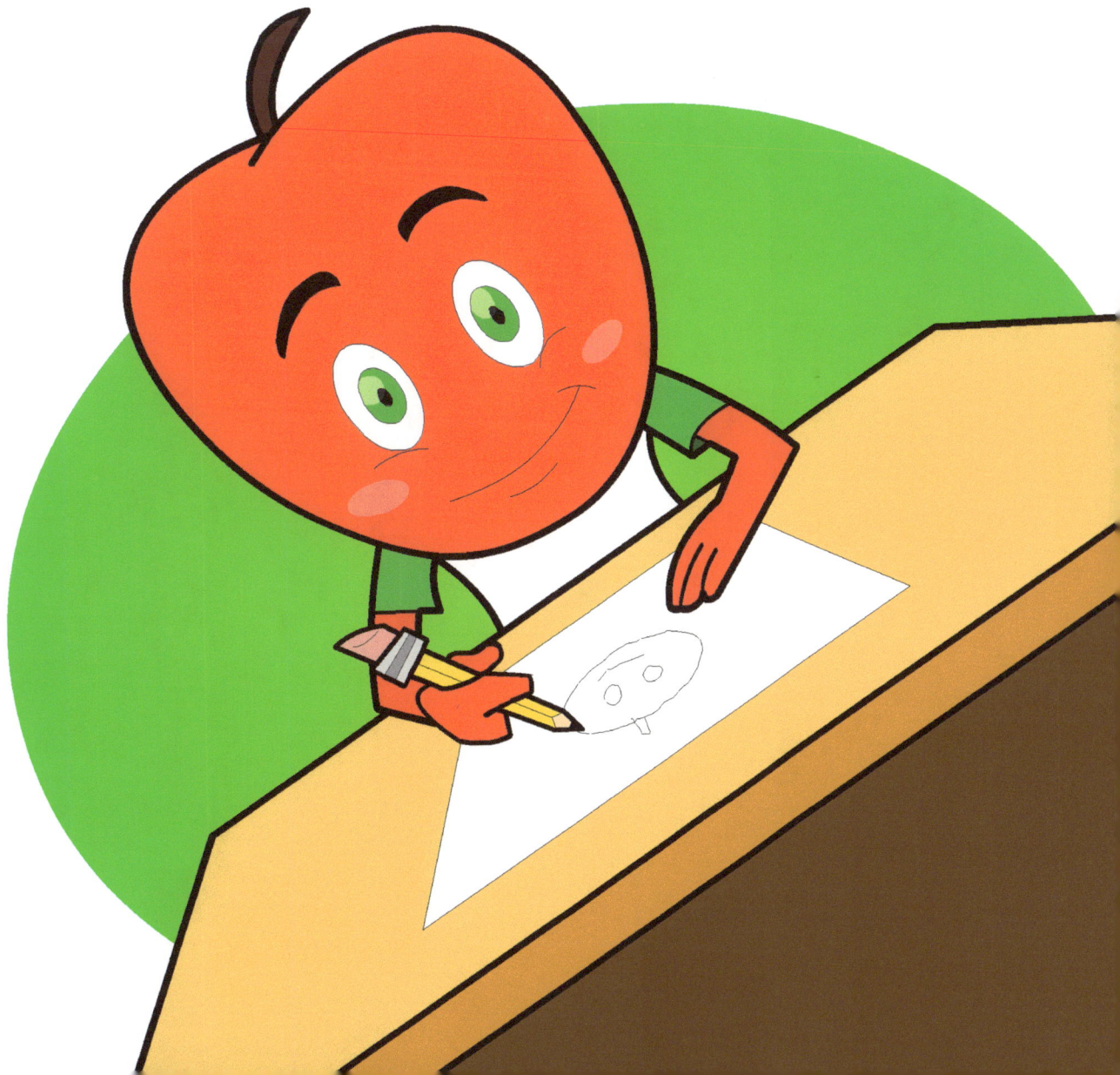

Carl
said with great passion,
"I am special because
I can write
with my left hand!"

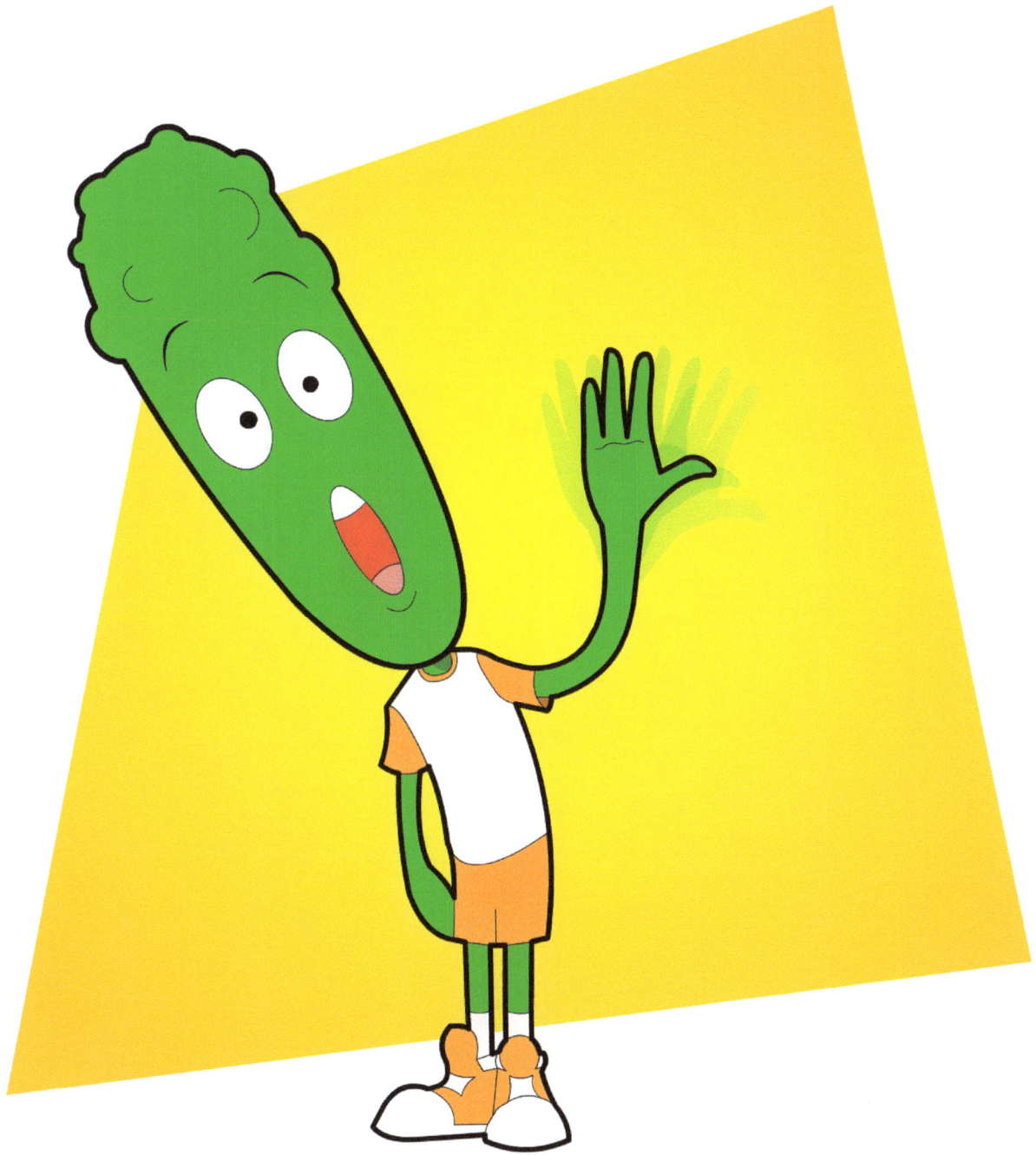

Peter proudly said,

"I am special because

I don't smell bad!"

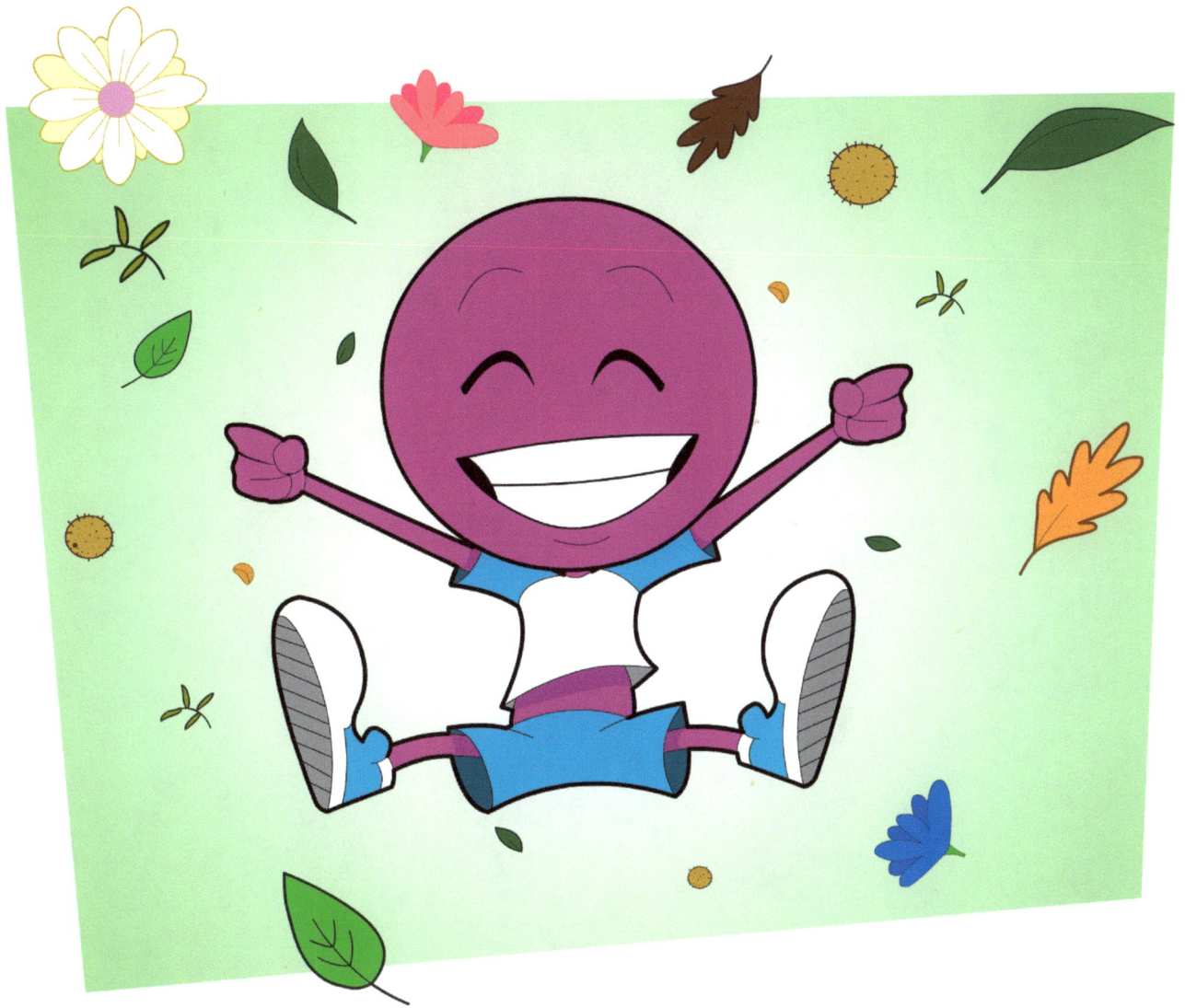

Bobby said,
"I am special because I can cook."

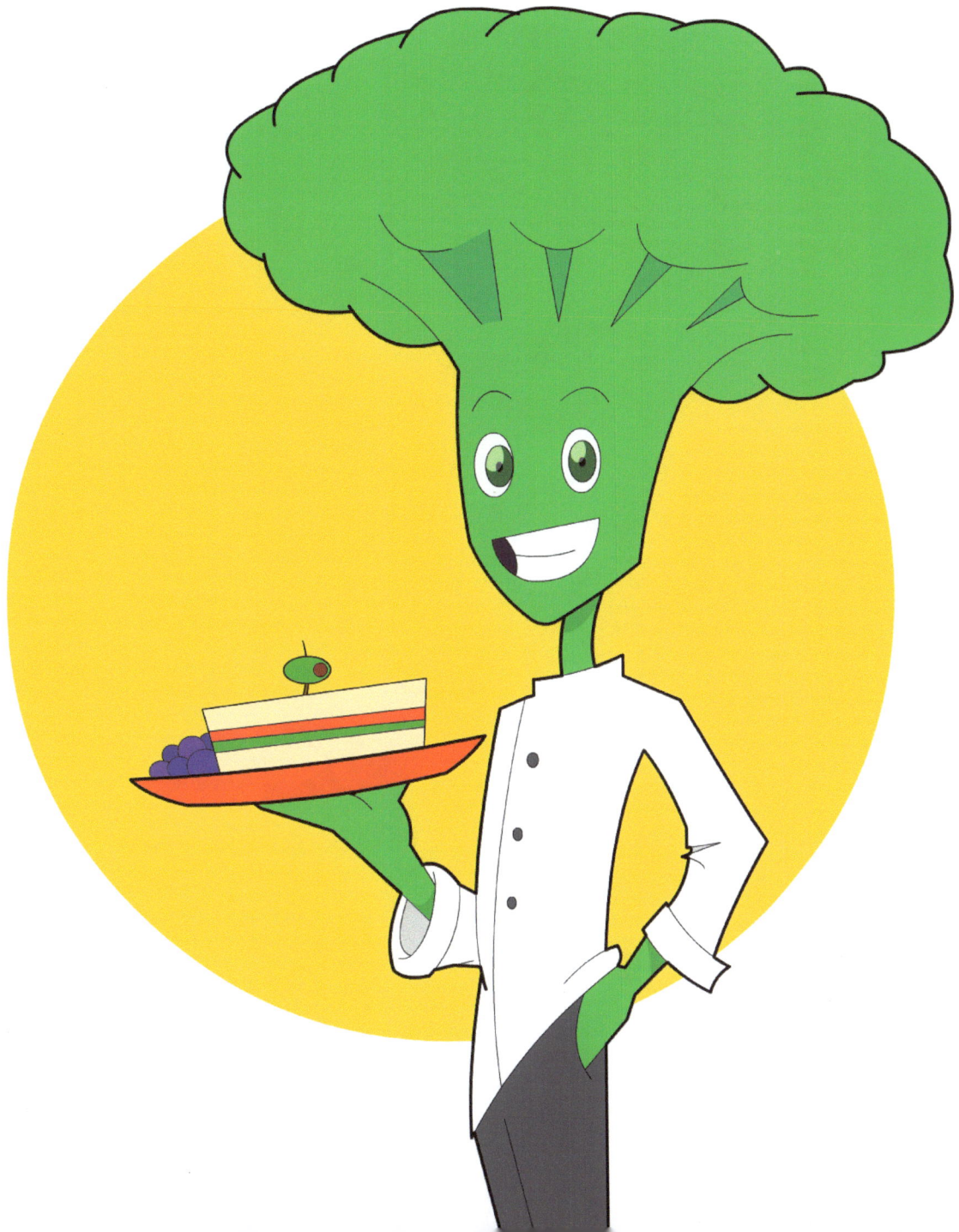

Pricilla said,
"I am special because
I can make music."

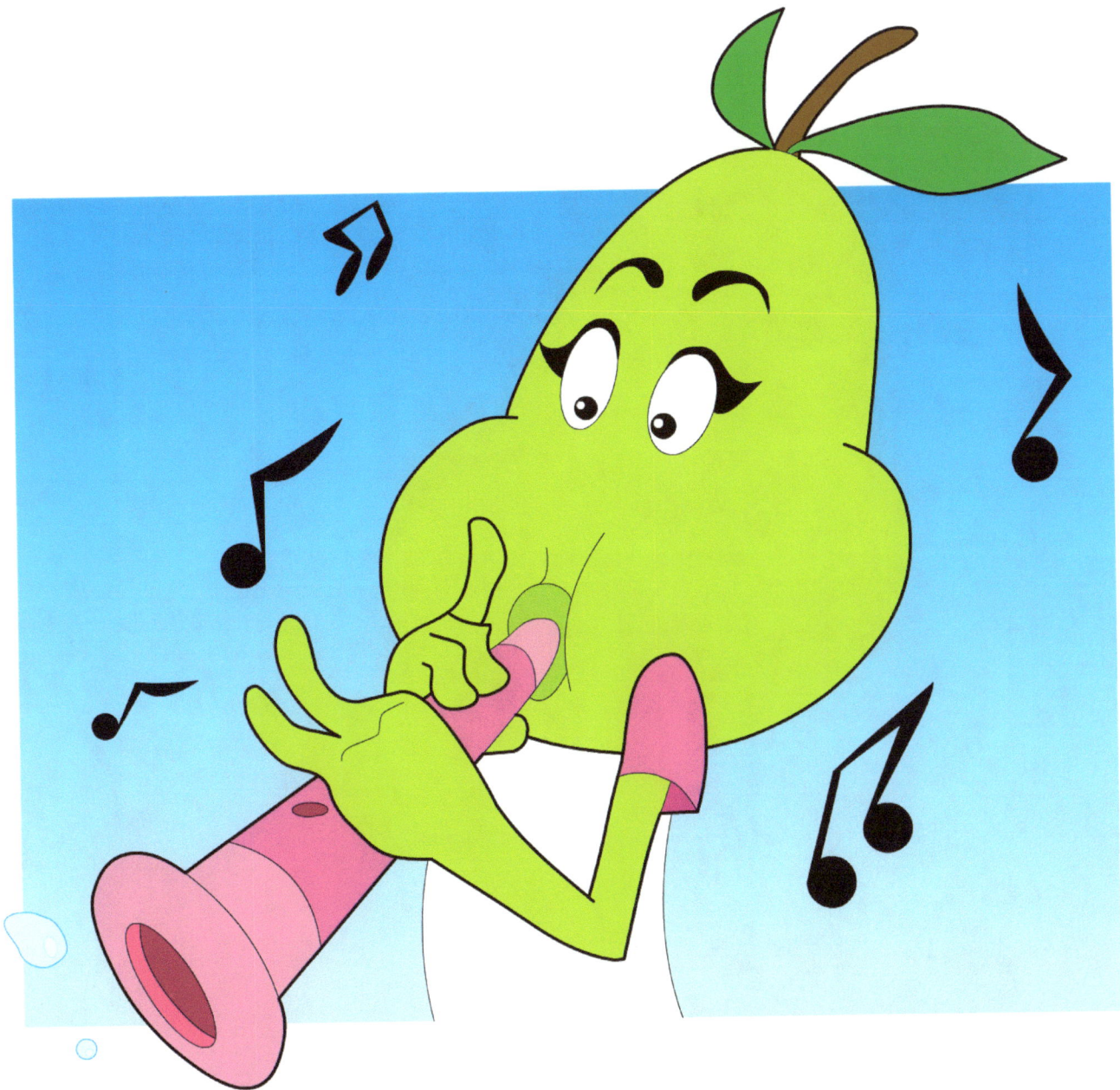

Zoey said,
"I am special because
I can dance."

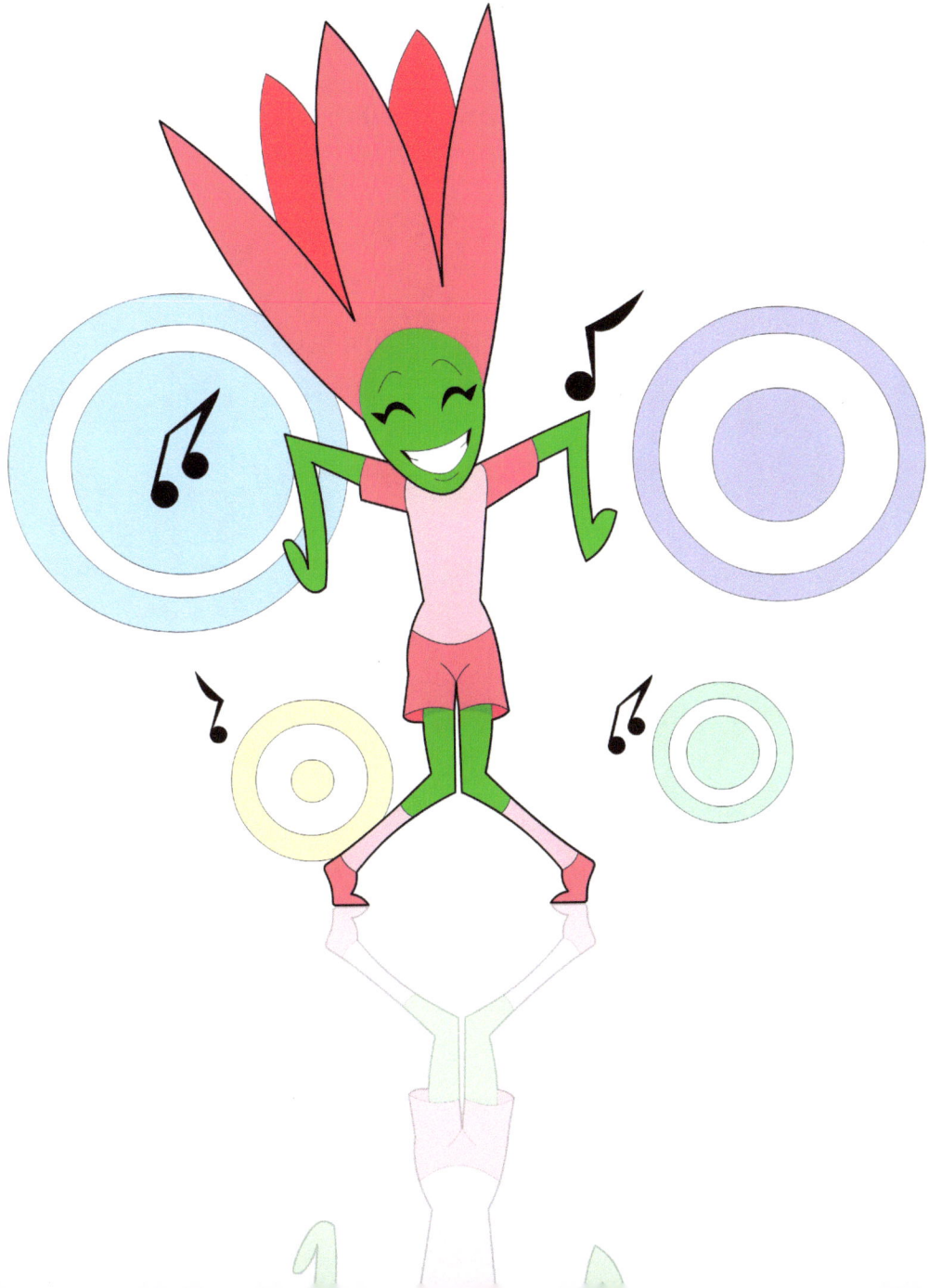

Sammie said,
"I am special because
I have style."

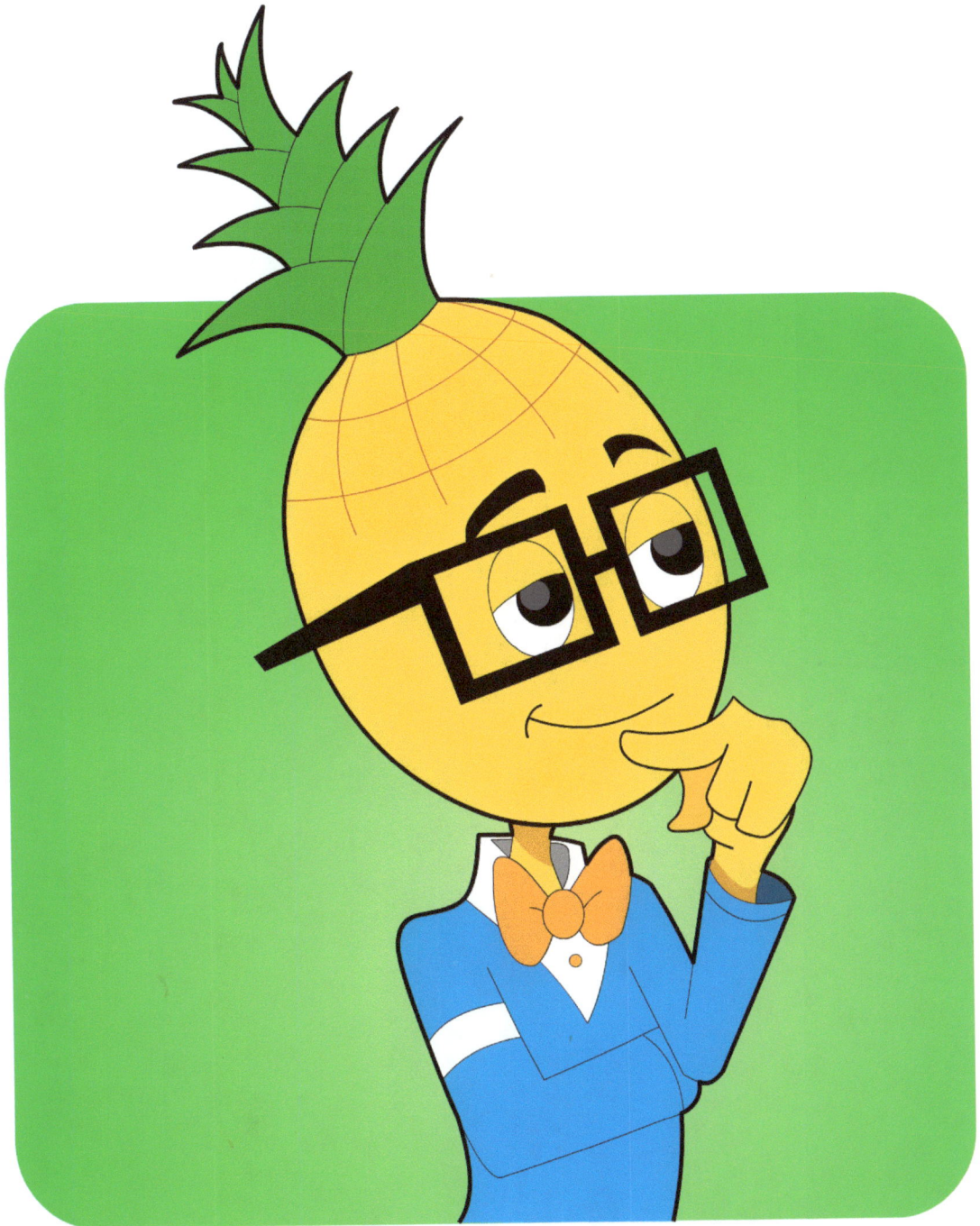

Oskar said,
"I am special because
I am a hard worker."

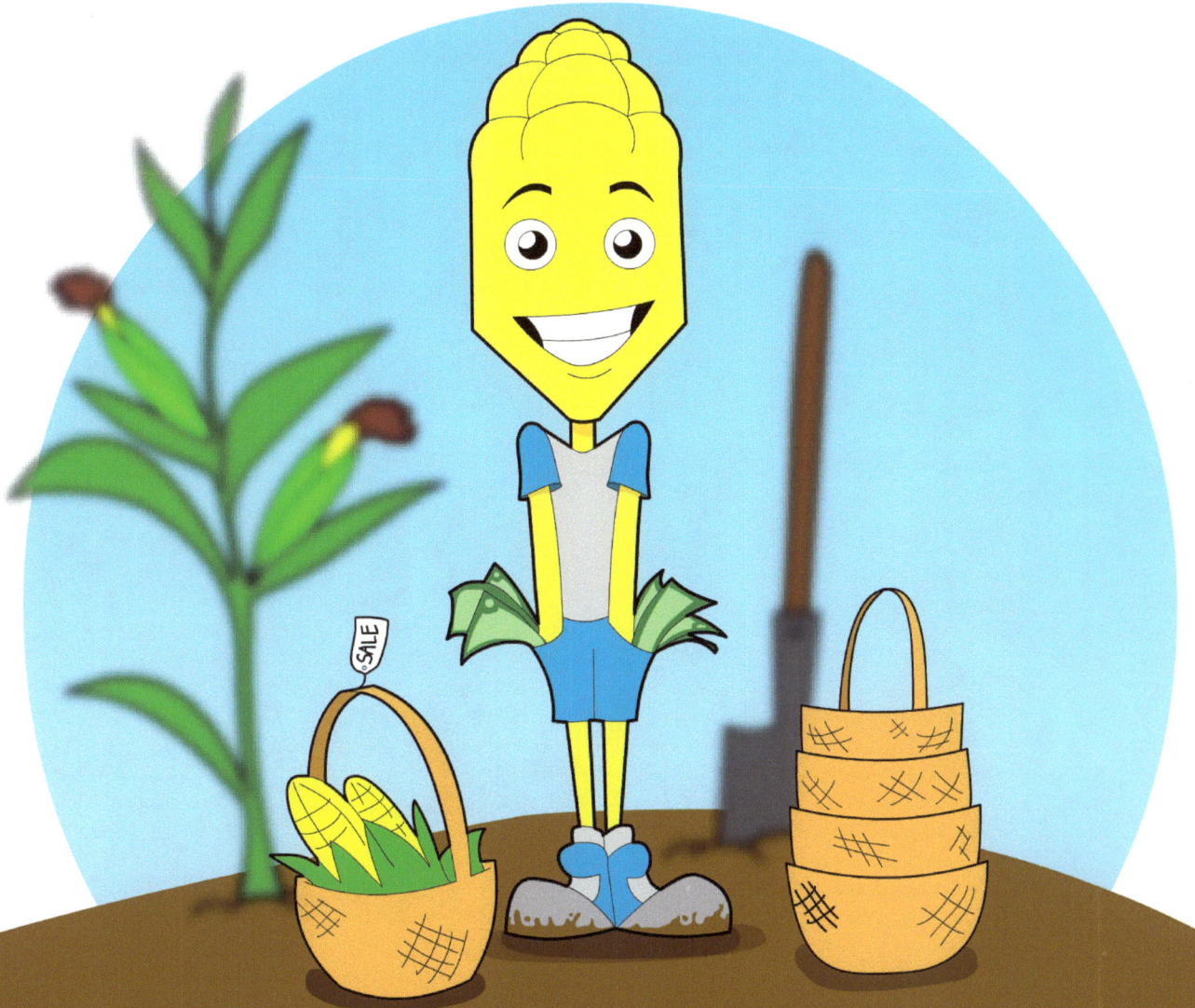

Sara said,
"I am special because

I'm nice
to everyone."

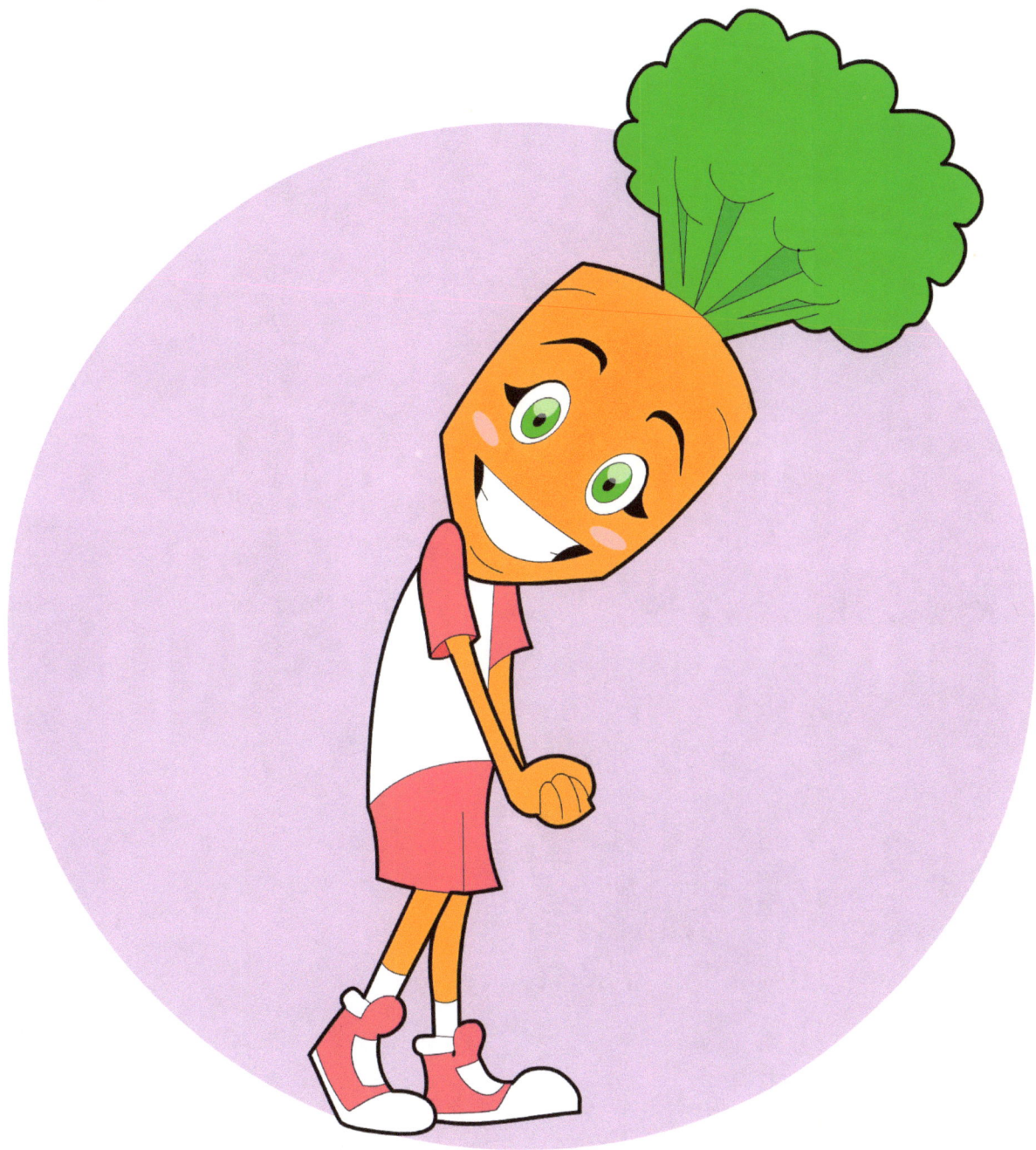

Lenard said,
"I am special because
I never give up."

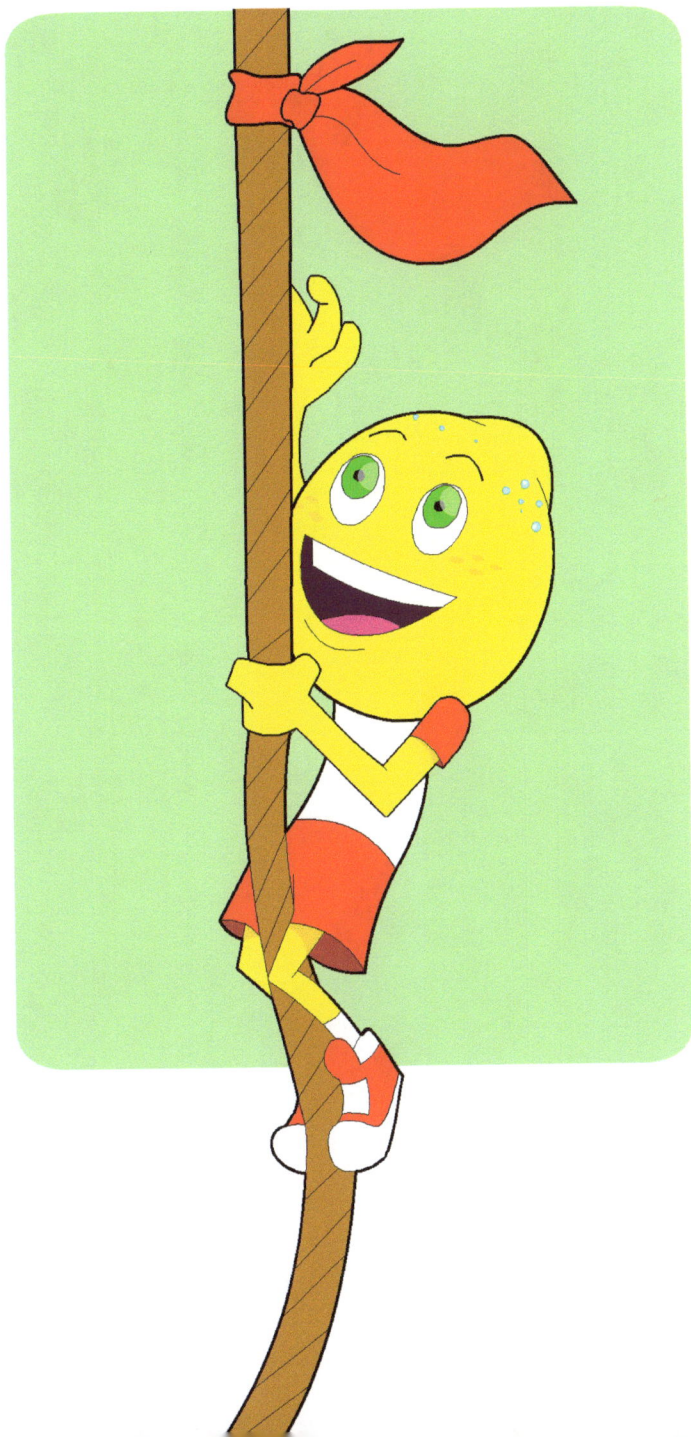

Blake said,
"I am special because
I'm good at sports."

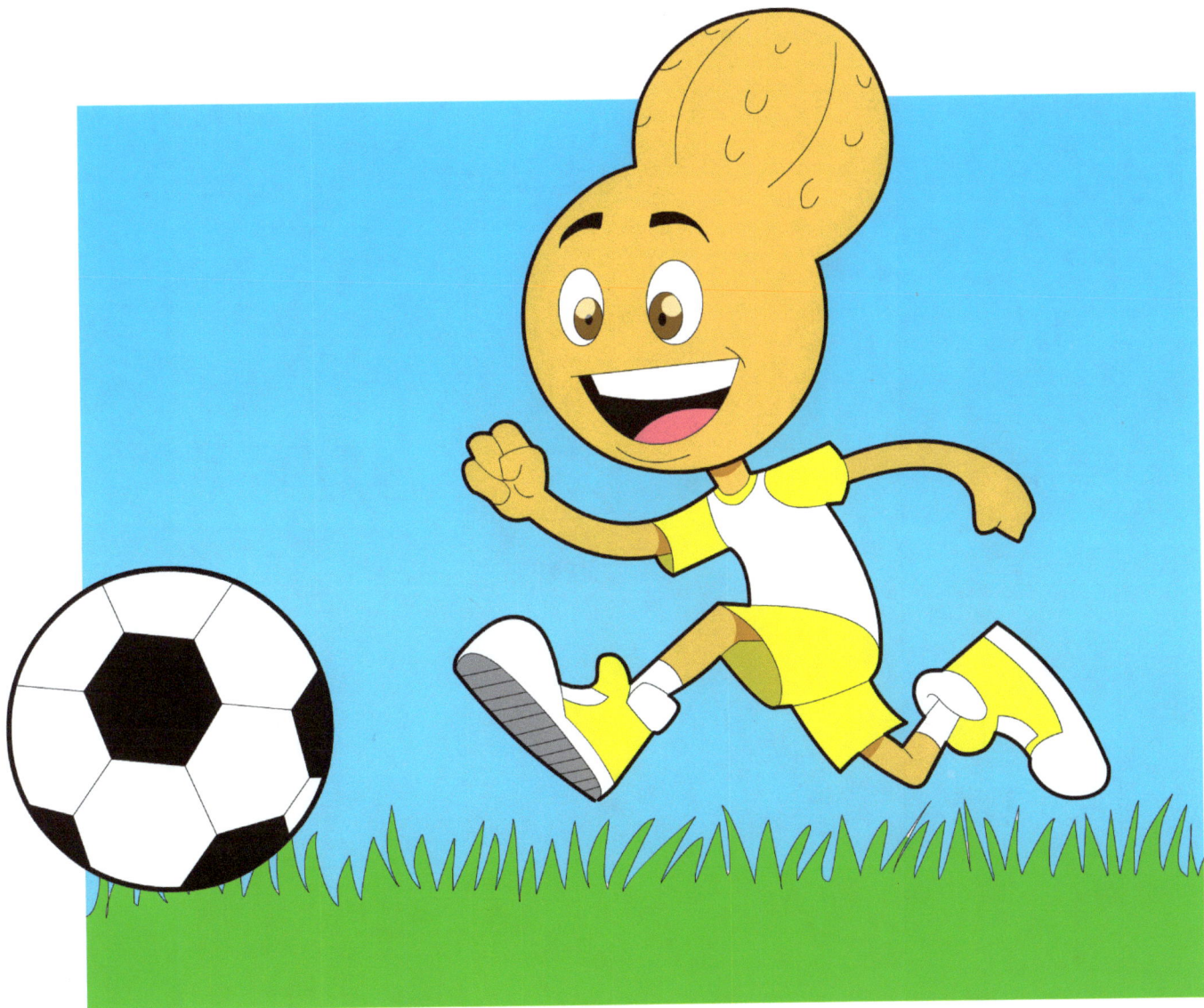

James said,
"I am special because
I love to read."

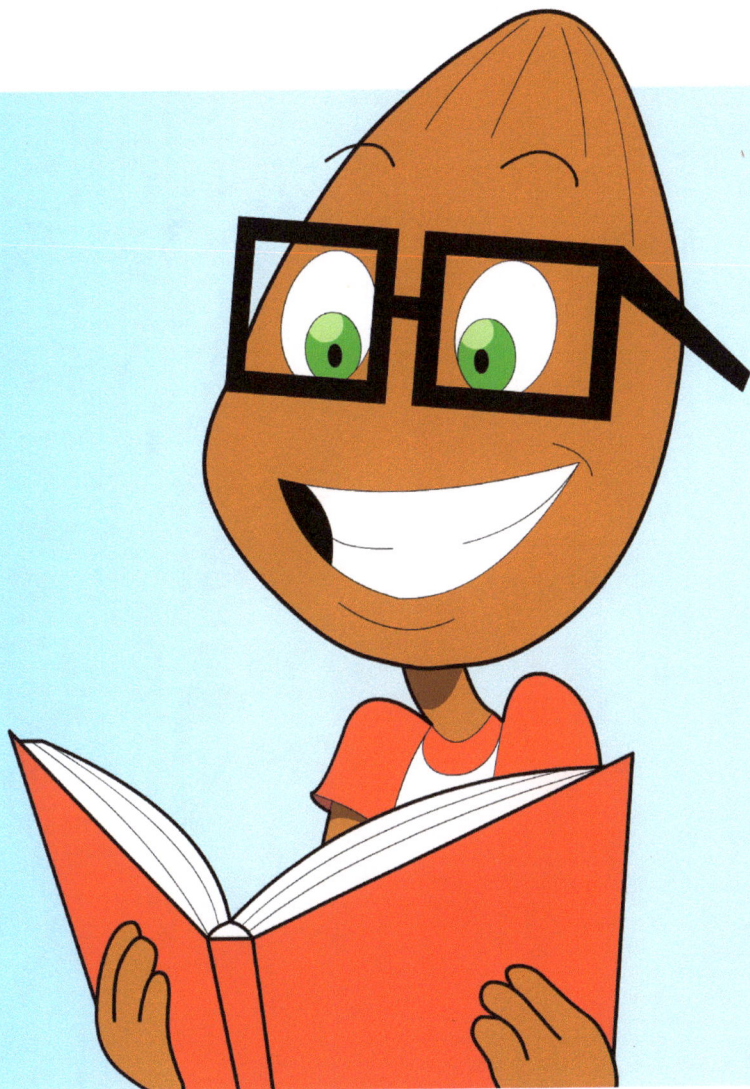

Gloria said,
"I am special because
I can sing."

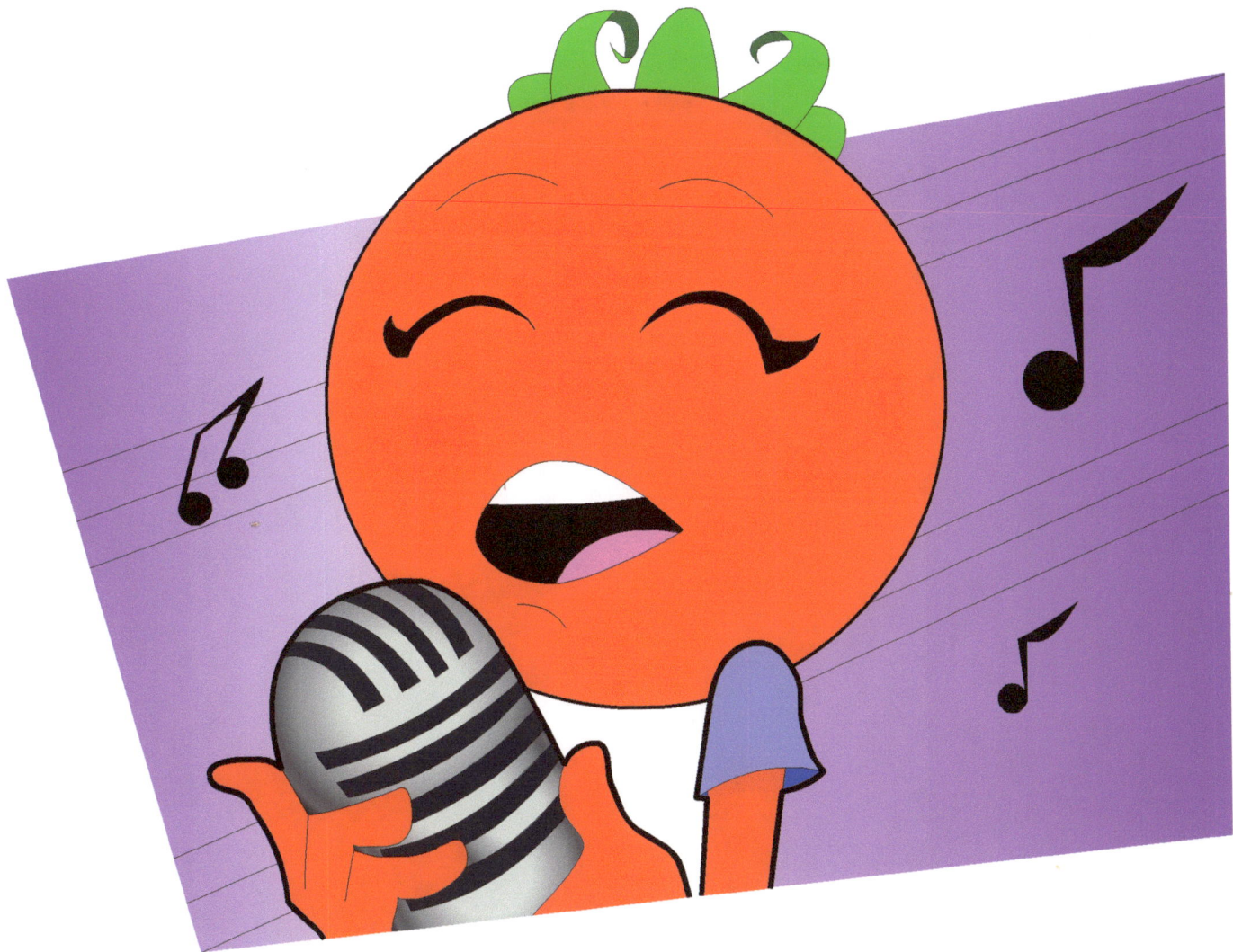

As for me,
I am special because

I have people in my life
that love me.

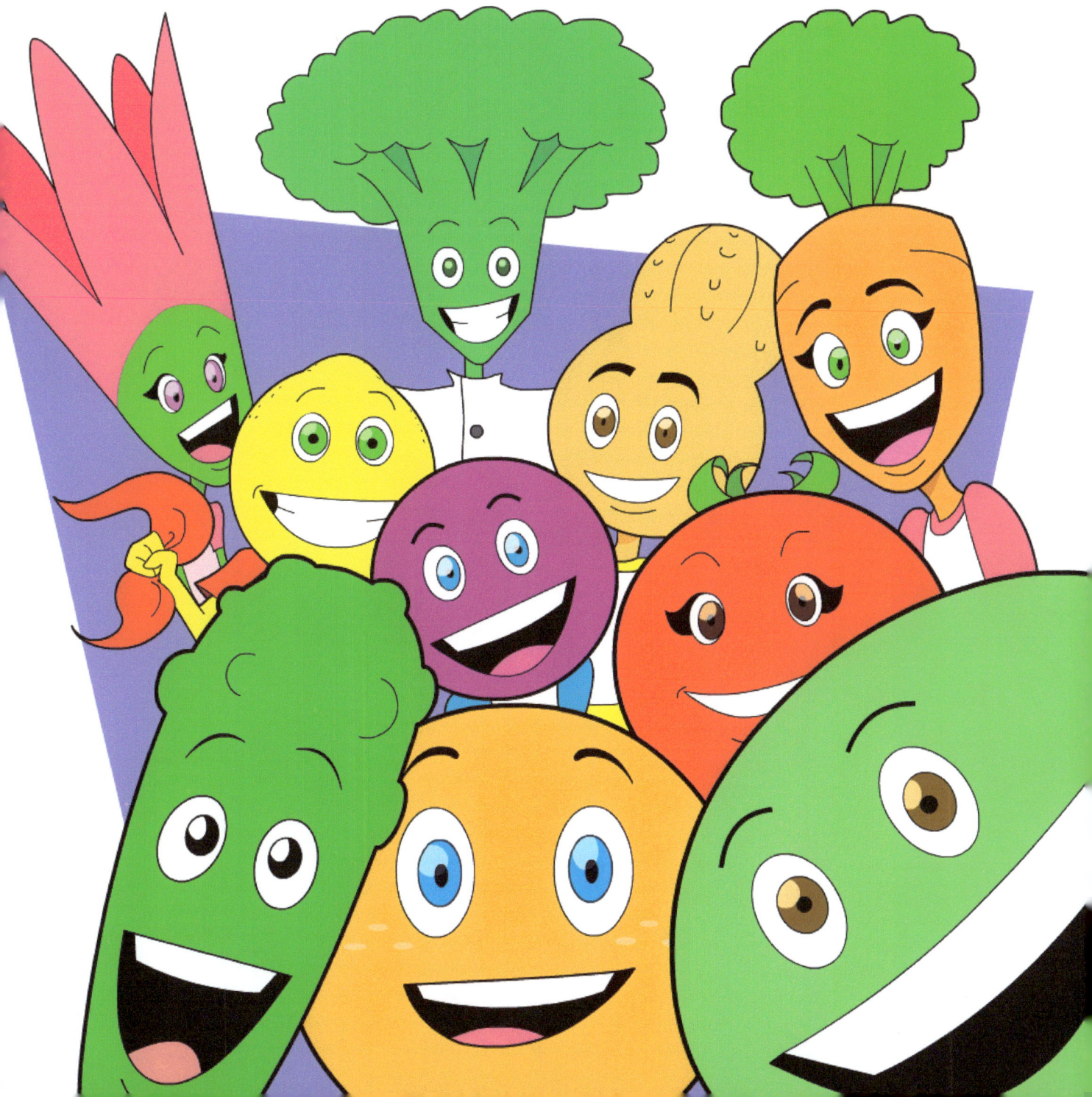

www.ingramcontent.com/pod-product-compliance
Lightning Source LLC
Chambersburg PA
CBHW061137030426
42334CB00003B/69